I0441614

Folk Remedies for the Modern Age

Anthony Canelo

Copyright © 2013 Anthony Canelo
All rights reserved.

ISBN: 1482618648
ISBN 13: 9781482618648

Library of Congress Control Number: 2013903829
CreateSpace Independent Publishing Platform,
North Charleston, SC

Other Books By Anthony Canelo

The Nature Pyramid

The Seven Fundamentals of Longevity

Marriage, Incarceration, Death, Religion, and Patience

Sleep: The Great Medicine

Creationships

Slowness Gives Wholeness

The Complete Compact Guide to Disaster Survival

Revival of the Fittest: The Prime Material for Human Health and Wisdom

The Revival of the Fittest: A Manual to Change the World

Self Determination: The Strategy to Master Addiction in America

Why I Wrote This Book

I wrote *Folk Remedies for the Modern Age* with the sustainability of your home and health in mind. How can vinegar, baking soda, hydrogen peroxide, sea salt, raw bee products, olive oil, colloidal silver, castor oil, glycothymoline, a black scarf, activated charcoal, and a high-frequency violet ray improve your health and well-being? Perhaps the ordinary nature of these items escapes our curiosity. You probably have most of them in your home now.

Originally, I wrote a short pamphlet on folk remedies for my guests at the Phoenix Institute. When I saw friends and family who had consulted with me at my office use these items on a daily basis, I became inspired to write this book. Now when one friend has a terrible stomachache, she ingests activated charcoal before resting. If another has incessant cravings for sugar, he drinks a teaspoon of apple cider vinegar. If another has an outbreak of herpes on the face, he uses a violet ray to help bring the condition back under control. If my mother suffers acid indigestion, she massages castor oil on her chest and neck. They've never been disappointed. Neither will you.

How many people do you know who walk into a beautiful forest and say, "You know, this is disappointing me; we need to cut all this down"? Nobody. In fact, many indigenous cultures know how to use every part of the tree itself, from root bark to outer leaf to branch. Most Americans do not know how to use what they already possess. They shop for items they don't need, while what they do need rests at home on dusty shelves.

Today, people knowingly consume polluted food. Health care costs are rising. Standards of living are falling. The writing is on the wall. You have only to look at the obese one-third of the American population[2]

1 **Overweight and Obesity,** Center for Disease Control, http://www.cdc.gov/obesity/data/adult.html, updated August 13, 2012.

to see that things are way out of control. But I love simple answers. *Folk Remedies for the Modern Age* will share fast, natural, and practical ways to support your health and healing. Don't you think it's time people took some of their health power back? I do.

Have you ever wondered why hydrogen peroxide was the most popular health-promoting product of the late nineteenth century? Have you wondered why activated charcoal is used in the water and air purification systems in submarines and space shuttles? Think about these things as you mark and turn the pages of this book. I would love to hear my readers tell me that they use all of the natural items I use on a regular basis; there is a sacred quality to learning more about simple, everyday things.

So , if you are looking to improve your health and vitality, increase your energy and concentration so that the person in the mirror is the best you that you can be, then this book will help you do that by discovering what has been sitting *behind* the mirror for all these years. Please have a seat, brew some hot tea, and get cozy. Your journey begins now.

As with any serious health condition, it is best to consult with your regular health care practitioner and/or medical doctor as you progress on your healing journey.

We all have a part to play. This is mine. I hope you enjoy.

To your health,

Anthony J. Canelo

"Thus the Sage rules,
By stilling the minds and opening hearts
By filling bellies and strengthening bones..."

—LAO TZU

FOLK REMEDIES FOR THE MODERN AGE

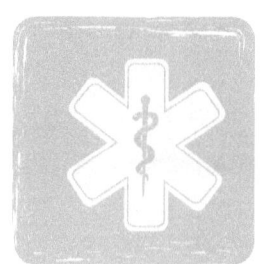

VINEGAR

The Son of Wine

Ryan Monay is twenty-four years old. He came to see me because of his uncontrollable cravings for breads, sodas, and sugary foods. I introduced him to the benefits of using vinegar in his daily diet. He immediately started to use apple cider vinegar and red wine vinegar on a regular and consistent basis to control his food cravings. Miraculously, his skin, physique, and body odor improved within one month. Ryan now understands that both apple cider vinegar and red wine vinegar contain large amounts of nutrients that the body needs. These help to satiate his hunger. He also understands that the acidic properties of these vinegars assist in the digestion of foods. For appetite suppression, I suggested he drink at least four tablespoons of apple cider vinegar or red wine vinegar each day, twenty minutes before or after meals. Since visiting the Phoenix Institute, he swears that a little apple cider vinegar each day controls his food cravings.

Vinegar Is a Superfood

Vinegar means "sour wine." It is actually an impure, diluted solution of acetic acid obtained through fermentation beyond the alcohol stage. The medicinal properties of vinegar are largely untold. Used properly, it is a superfood. Raw apple cider vinegar and red wine vinegar have more nutritional value than any other kind of vinegar.

Your body needs good acids to function properly. Apple cider vinegar contains large amounts of potassium, enzymes, calcium, iron, magnesium, beta-carotene, catechins, flavonoids, quercetin, and resveratrol. Its beneficial acids help digest foods, dissolve fat, and suppress appetite while still safely maintaining the body's alkaline/acid balance. When processed properly, vinegar can contain large amounts of beneficial bacteria, which help the immune system oxidize foreign pathogens and the digestive acids oxidize foods. In other words, it is a good acid. This adds to its healing powers.

During the Civil War, traveling soldiers used apple cider vinegar to prevent scurvy or vitamin C deficiency. The samurai would drink a water and vinegar dilution because they said it gave them energy. Aside from a well-balanced nutritional profile, the magic of vinegar lies in its acidic nature. Roman soldiers added sea salt to vinegar and water, claiming it an energy tonic. Vinegar and sea salt in water make a wonderful blend that can increase performance and mental energy. The acids in vinegar help to break down the sea salt for digestion, easing assimilation of its mineral content.

During the SARS (Severe Acute Respiratory Syndrome) outbreak of early 2003, the Chinese government had to strictly regulate the rising price of vinegar.[2] Why? Because any form of vinegar, if used properly, can help clean and detoxify the respiratory system. Gargling vinegar for just for a few moments, then swallowing it, works most effectively.

---

2 Cal Orey, *The Healing Powers of Vinegar: A Complete Guide to Nature's Most Remarkable Remedy* (New York City, Kensington Publishing Corporation) 2009 page 69.

It's All About Balance

The body needs an acid/alkali balance. Any imbalance will diminish the body's ability to strengthen and build protein. A low carbohydrate/ high alkaline diet may be a fad today, but after the initial grace period of healing, an over-alkaline diet can actually lead to dangerously low levels of body fat, diminished brain power, memory loss, the promotion of certain parasites, and even cancer. Parasites and certain cancers can survive in an over-alkaline environment, yet those same cancers and parasites could never survive in a body with a consistently balanced pH. I suggest a high alkaline diet only for people who are over-acidic. I recommend checking your pH regularly and eating a pH-balanced diet. To testing your pH, you can purchase pH tester strips online or at your local health food store. The ideal pH for your saliva and urine is 6.4.

Dr. C's Sleepy Time Tonic and Vitamin Lemonade

As a health coach, I recommend you incorporate the following folk remedies into your regular health regime. The first one uses apple cider vinegar to foster restorative deep sleep. I believe deep sleep is the most important key to maintaining physical health. Most people do not sleep deep enough. The truly restorative process—called healing— begins only when we fall, and stay, asleep. So it is wise to take care of your sleep, first and foremost. To accomplish this, bring filtered water to a boil. Combine one teaspoon of honey with three teaspoons of bee pollen. Then add four teaspoons of apple cider vinegar. I often make myself one or two cups of this delicious apple cider vinegar, which I call my Sleepy Time Tonic.

Conversely, if I want to liven up my day, I use a different sort of recipe for apple cider vinegar. I juice three whole lemons, add two tablespoons of apple cider vinegar or red wine vinegar, then add an appropriate amount of distilled or filtered water. I pour this simple lemonade into a glass pitcher and drink it throughout the day. I call it Dr. C's Vitamin Lemonade.

Did You Know?

According to Pliny, a Roman scholar, Cleopatra wagered her husband Marc Antony that she could eat a meal that would cost a million sestertius (an old Roman coin). The bet seemed absurd because one person can only consume so much at one sitting. At mealtime, the queen simply dropped a million sestertius' worth of pearls into a glass of vinegar. She put aside her "meal" while the rest of the food was prepared. Before she took her first bite, the queen swallowed the pearls dissolved in vinegar. Cleopatra understood the properties of vinegar very well indeed![3]

In 1000 AD, the queen of Hungary used an apple cider vinegar-based tonic on her skin. It suited the cosmetic needs of medieval European royalty due to its astringent and antiseptic qualities.[4]

And Even More Surprising

Nobel Prize winner Dr. Alexis Carrel (1912–1940) did an experiment to keep cells from a chicken heart alive, reproducing new cells for twenty-eight years. He kept these cells alive by removing cellular waste accumulated in the cells (detoxification) and feeding the cells a nutrient-rich solution.[5] Guess what main ingredient he used in his nutrient-rich solution: apple cider vinegar!

So, what are the other uses for which vinegar has been recognized in ancient times?

1. Hippocrates used a blend of pepper, raw honey, and vinegar for feminine disorders.
2. The Egyptians used vinegar to treat mushroom poisoning, worms in the ears, severe loss of appetite, and gangrene.

---

3 Ibid, page 13.
4 http://mountainroseblog.com/queen-hungarys-water/
Queen of Hungary's Water. Mountain Rose Blog posted on 21 March 2012
5 Ibid.

3. In medieval times, vinegar with rosemary and lavender was used to treat unease of the stomach and the brain.
4. For over one thousand years, raw honey and vinegar have been used to remove phlegm and treat coughs.
5. The Royal Society of London used vinegar as a gargle for mouth and throat infections and on the scalp for dandruff.
6. Compresses of vinegar and water have been used for centuries to help burns heal more quickly.

Here are some easy ways for you to add vinegar to your diet:

- Add red wine vinegar to hot pepper and sea salt. Shake well every day for ten days. After ten days, you will have your own hot sauce.
- Add raw apple cider vinegar to baby carrots for a knockout beta-carotene-rich meal.
- Add red wine vinegar to cinnamon powder or liquid vitamin C for a synergistic effect in metabolizing vitamin C.
- Take one or two tablespoons of raw apple cider or red wine vinegar after meals to help with digestion. For larger meals, or if you are overweight, take three to nine tablespoons.

If you remember why red apple cider and red wine vinegar are good for you, then you will be able to come up with your own ideas for incorporating vinegar into your diet:

- Enhances the immune system
- Fights deadly food bacteria
- Prevents infection
- Kills viruses
- Aids digestion

Baking Soda
A powerful addition to your medicine cabinet

Another great addition to your health arsenal is baking soda. Why? Well, naturally occurring bicarbonates help to alkalize the entire body, or in other words, buffer acids. Our body makes these bicarbonates, as well as other substances, to keep its mineral ratios in proper balance. A healthy newborn baby has a balanced acid-to-alkali ratio or *pH*. Every living organism on Earth is designed to have a balanced acid-to-alkali ratio within its body.[6]

The Importance of Being Alkaline

Unfortunately, many of our modern-day habits contribute to excessive acid ratios in the body. Some of the great culprits include sodas, excessive amounts of alcohol, artificial or high-sugar diets, and stress. Baking soda helps to neutralize excessive acid in the body. In particular, it can help neutralize excessive carbonic acid. Carbonic acid, a critical component to life, can easily build up when a person is unable to exhale

---

6 Even our farm soils are ideally balanced according to their pH.

fully. Habitual shallow breathing can trap carbon dioxide in the lungs, where it can produce excess carbonic acid and become dangerous to the body. In fact, many people receive respiration in the emergency rooms at hospitals because they typically inhale 20 percent oxygen from the air but exhale only 18 percent, indicating that their bodies are unable to process carbon dioxide, which could prevent effective treatment. Nature has designed a backup system for shallow breathers, however. The kidneys have the ability to secrete bicarbonates in order to neutralize excessive acid build up.

Baking Soda Health Tips: Deep Breathing and Soaking

To properly use baking soda, it is important to understand the importance of deep breathing. One teaspoon of aluminum-free baking soda in a glass of water can utterly change the body's mineral ratios, and it costs only pennies a day. When you combine this drink with five minutes of deep, relaxed breathing, the results are extraordinarily soothing.

Some Other Health and Beauty Uses for Baking Soda

If you are holistically health-minded and want to incorporate more natural remedies into your life, here are some additional helpful suggestions.

To Remove Odors:

- Place an open box of baking soda in your refrigerator, under your sinks, in garbage cans—anywhere you'd like to reduce odors.
- Sprinkle it as a powder under your armpits.

As a Solution:

- Use four tablespoons in one quart of warm water, or up to half a box in a full bathtub, to alkalize bathwater, work as a disinfectant, or relieve sunburn pain and itching.
- Drink two teaspoons dissolved in filtered water to help pass kidney stones.
- For bad breath, add a dash of baking soda to a glass of water and use as a gargle.

As a Sprinkle:

- Apply lightly to a damp cloth or sponge to clean and disinfect countertops, windows, and other surfaces.

Remember, baking soda is beneficial because of these four important characteristics:

- It has a soft, crystalline molecular structure that does not stain or scar.
- It has the ability to neutralize acidity.
- It is a leavening agent.
- It absorbs many odors.

By The Way: Dr. Mark Sircus has written many books and made YouTube videos championing the use of baking soda for the treatment of cancer.[7]

---

7 Mark Sircus, *Sodium Bicarbonate - A Full Medical Review,* International Medical Veritas Association (2010).

Hydrogen Peroxide
A Must-Have for the Home

For its sheer health benefits, hydrogen peroxide is arguably the most important thing to have in your home. I recommend having at least two or three bottles on hand. According to the famous German chemist, Dr. Koenig, the average person weighing 160 pounds is composed of 90 pounds of oxygen and 14 pounds of hydrogen, respectively. If you search for a way to modulate and balance these two utterly critical elements found in all forms of life, you will discover a tonic. That tonic is called hydrogen peroxide. Any form of hydrogen peroxide is useful to keep you in good health; however, the most common dilution for external use is typically 3 percent. Food-grade hydrogen peroxide is usually 12 percent or higher.

Before the pharmaceutical industry gained market power over natural approaches to health, hydrogen peroxide was the most widely sold health product in the United States. Duke University began studies using hydrogen peroxide intravenously and topically on ill or healing patients. They found hydrogen peroxide tremendously beneficial to the heart and nervous system; in fact, they found that it benefited the whole body. However, the American Medical Association shut down the study, and support of hydrogen peroxide by the medical community has since dwindled

The Body's Little Cleaners

Hydrogen peroxide is a naturally occurring chemical within the human body. It is processed with the help of vitamin C and coenzyme Q10 (CoQ10). The more of these nutrients you are able to absorb, the better your ability to synthesize hydrogen peroxide on your own to clean your body. Hydrogen peroxide within the body functions primarily as a detergent. Along with oxygen, nitric oxide, and antioxidants, I like to think of hydrogen peroxide molecules as the little cleaners of every cell in the body, cleaning both cells and cell fluids. Most importantly, hydrogen peroxide oxygenates as it cleans. The process of cellular cleansing is sometimes called oxygenation.

Scientists don't dispute the fact that toxic, dirty cells accelerate all forms of imbalance in our bodies. How can chemicals or pharmaceutical products containing toxic substances that block molecular channels in the body, cause allergies, or keep you up at night, be good for you? Hardly any positive side effects exist from most chemical drugs. Do yourself a favor: whether it's a hydrogen peroxide mouthwash, footbath, or hand soak, help yourself by cleaning your cells with hydrogen peroxide.

How Natural Is Hydrogen Peroxide?

Rainwater is 1 percent hydrogen peroxide. That's why it is so useful in disinfecting and properly oxygenating soils. Without hydrogen peroxide in our rainwater, our crops would wither and die before we could eat them. In our bodies as well as in nature, a sophisticated form of oxygen – called ozone – is often found with hydrogen peroxide, which produces beneficial chemicals in our bodies, called reactive oxygen species. We are only beginning to understand what our own immune systems—our T-cells, white blood cells, and macrophages (soldiers on the ground, if you will)—use to combat invaders and excess free radicals. Yes, they use different forms of oxygen to kill pathogens. In effect, they breathe health back into us. At the Phoenix Institute, we use hydrogen peroxide for hand and foot soaks, at times using an ozone generator to assist the cleansing process. The results have been fantastic: in a number of cases, varicose veins have disappeared within a few weeks and pain in the joints has lessened in only a few minutes.

Health Uses

I cannot overemphasize the benefits of using hydrogen peroxide as part of your daily health care routine. You will be able to ward off infection before it can take hold and find almost immediate gains in your health and well-being.

Hydrogen peroxide gargle routine: Gargle four to six times a day before meals, or forty-five minutes after meals for two weeks. Gargling with hydrogen peroxide oxygenates the blood, ears, eyes, and throat.

Internal use: Only use hydrogen peroxide for internal purposes if it is food-grade hydrogen peroxide. It is a fantastic free radical scavenger, and an antiviral, antibiotic, and antifungal agent. Before using hydrogen peroxide internally, make sure you consult first with your doctor or health care practitioner.

Hydrogen peroxide hand/foot soaks: To a basin or tub, add the following ingredients:

- 20 parts water
- 1 part hydrogen peroxide
- 1 teaspoon salt (Recommended salts: Epsom salt, sea salt, common table salt)

Soak for twenty minutes

You may also try stronger solutions, such as one part hydrogen peroxide and ten parts water, or one part hydrogen peroxide and fifteen parts water.

For chronic and sub-acute conditions, such as arthritis, gout, Hashimoto's disease or high blood pressure, hydrogen peroxide foot soaks should be taken daily, but no less than four or five days a week.

Support Your Health

Household Uses: Support your health with substances that actually keep your body and home fresh, and not with industrial chemicals that pose as household cleaners. Hydrogen peroxide can function as an effective household cleaner, especially when teamed up with baking soda and vinegar. Listed below are excellent examples of household uses of hydrogen peroxide.

1. A large spray bottle of hydrogen peroxide and alcohol (1:1) is the best disinfectant money can buy. You can use it to wipe down tables, computer keyboards, steering wheels, sickrooms, etc. Add a few drops of lavender to this mixture for a delightful and healthful scent.
   a. Use the spray to sterilize and eliminate shower and soil mold or mildew.
   b. Spray the inside of toilet bowls as a disinfectant.
2. Use it to water plants: mix one ounce of 3 percent hydrogen peroxide to one hundred ounces of water.
3. Clean pesticides off of conventional produce.

Remember that hydrogen peroxide will break down when exposed to light, so store it in opaque containers.

Sea Salt
Don't Be Home Without It

Human beings have a long history with salt. Ancient Egyptians used it as a religious offering. Ancient Romans used it as a method of payment. In fact, this is where the word *salary* originated. Salt (or sodium) is very important for human health. It cleans the lymphatic system, helps the body to retain water, balances calcium, alkalizes the body, and tones the muscles and skin. Salt is native to every body of water, every kind of soil, every plant, and every animal on Earth. In fact, the average 160-pound person has close to three ounces of sodium within him or her. Organic sodium is always best, coming from natural foods, such as sea veggies, kale, or olives. Inorganic sodium, however, is a ready and capable substitute, provided that you do not have too much sodium in your diet to begin with.

These days, sea salt is a renowned health food commodity. Many types exist; I prefer either brown or pink sea salt. Dead Sea salt has over twenty-five major minerals in it, while typical sea salt contains closer to three. In a world where many believe that water will become the most valuable resource on the planet, salt will inevitably rank much higher in importance than it does today. Perhaps in the future, salt might once again be used as a currency.

We Came from the Sea

Our bodies share an almost identical mineral content with ocean water. When we ingest sea salt, the bacteria in our intestines break down these soft salt rocks and make them ready for use by the body.[8] A little sea salt will go a long way in a glass of water, together with vinegar, to treat mineral deficiencies.

Health and Beauty Tips

Sea salt is widely available, and so it is ideal for use at home or when traveling. I especially recommend it for keeping the mouth and breath clean. It has remarkable restorative qualities for those nights when you have had too much to eat or drink.

- **As a gargle**: Stir a half teaspoon of sea salt into an eight-ounce glass of warm water for sore throats.
- **To clean teeth**: Pulverize sea salt in a blender. Mix one part sea salt with two parts baking soda, then add water and apply to gums. This whitens teeth, helps remove plaque, and is healthy for the gums.
- **As a mouthwash**: Mix equal parts sea salt and baking soda in a glass of water to sweeten the breath.
- **As an eye bath**: Mix a half teaspoon of sea salt in a pint of water. Use the solution to bathe tired eyes.
- **To reduce eye puffiness**: Mix one teaspoon of sea salt in a pint of hot water. Soak pads in the solution and apply to puffy areas.
- **To relieve tired feet**: Soak aching feet in warm water with a handful of sea salt. Rinse in cool water.
- **To relieve bee stings**: If stung, immediately wet the spot and cover with sea salt to relieve the pain.
- **To treat mosquito and chigger bites**: Soak affected area in salt water, then apply a mixture of lard and sea salt.
- **To treat poison ivy**: Soak the exposed area in hot salt water to help relieve irritation.

---

8 Dr. Maynard Murray, *Sea Energy Agriculture* (Austin, Acres USA).

- **To relieve fatigue:** Soak for at least ten minutes in a tub of water with several handfuls of sea salt.

More Uses of Sea Salt

As a household cleaner, sea salt is an excellent and natural way to remove stains, deodorize smells, and brighten surfaces. I recommend sea salt for many home uses.

In the Kitchen

- **Stains on dishes**: Rub stain with sea salt (especially good for removing stubborn tea or coffee stains).
- **Ovens:** Sea salt and cinnamon will remove burnt food odors from ovens and stove burners. Sprinkle on spills while oven or burners are still hot. Let dry, then brush or wipe off the salted spots.
- **Refrigerators:** Use a sea salt and soda water solution to clean and sweeten the inside of your refrigerator.
- **Tarnished silverware**: Rub with sea salt before washing.
- **Copper pans**: Rub sea salt on stains, then scour with a cloth soaked in vinegar.
- **Coffee pots**: Fill with water, add four tablespoons of sea salt, then percolate or boil as usual.
- **Cutting boards:** Wash with soap and water, and then rub cutting boards with a damp cloth dipped in sea salt.
- **Brass:** Mix equal parts sea salt, flour, and vinegar to make a paste. Rub the paste on the brass item, and leave on for an hour or so. Clean with a soft cloth or brush and buff with a dry cloth.
- **Sink drains:** Pour a strong saltwater solution down the kitchen drain regularly to eliminate odors and keep grease from building up.
- **Extend broom life:** New brooms will wear longer if soaked in hot salt water before they are first used.

- **Restore sponges:** Wash sponges and then soak in cold salt water.
- **Onion odors:** Rub fingers or hands with sea salt that has been moistened with vinegar.
- **"Sweeten" containers:** Deodorize thermos bottles and other closed containers with sea salt.
- **Extinguish grease fires:** Toss sea salt on a grease fire to smother flames. Never use water; it will only spatter the burning grease.

For the Living Room

- **Wicker:** Scrub wicker furniture with a stiff brush moistened with warm salt water and allow it to dry in the sun.
- **Rugs:** You can remove some grease spots with a solution of one part sea salt and four parts alcohol. Rub firmly but carefully to avoid damaging the nap.
- **Rings from tables:** Remove rings left on tables from wet or hot dishes or glasses by rubbing a thin paste of salad oil and sea salt on the spot with your fingers. Let it stand an hour or two, and then wipe off.
- **Fish tanks:** Rub the inside of fish tanks with sea salt to remove hard water deposits, then rinse well before returning the fish to the tank. Do not use iodized salt.
- **Wine stains:** Blot the stain as much as possible and immediately cover the wine with salt, which will absorb the remaining wine. Rinse with cold water. When using on rugs, scrape up the salt from the rug and then vacuum the spot.

For Clothing

- **Perspiration stains**: Add four tablespoons of sea salt to one quart of hot water and sponge the fabric with the solution until stains disappear.
- **Bloodstains:** Soak the stained item in cold salt water, then launder in warm, soapy water and boil after the wash. Use only on cotton, linen, or other natural fibers.
- **Mildew or rust stains:** Moisten stains with a mixture of lemon juice and sea salt, then spread the item in the sun to bleach. Rinse and dry.
- **Brighten colors:** Wash colored curtains or washable fiber rugs in a saltwater solution to brighten the colors. Brighten faded rugs and carpets by rubbing them briskly with a cloth that has been dipped in a strong saltwater solution and wrung out. For yellowed cottons or linens, boil the yellowed items for one hour in a sea salt and baking soda solution (1:1).
- **Sticking irons:** Sprinkle a little sea salt on a piece of paper and run the hot iron over it to remove rough, sticky spots.
- **Bubbling suds:** If a washing machine bubbles over from too many suds, sprinkle salt on the suds to reduce them.

For Food

- **To improve coffee taste:** A pinch of sea salt in coffee will enhance the flavor and remove the bitter taste of overcooked coffee.
- **To improve the flavor of poultry:** Rub the fowl inside and out with sea salt before roasting.
- **To whip cream and egg whites:** Add a pinch of sea salt; cream will whip better, and egg whites will beat faster and higher.
- **To keep milk fresh:** Add a pinch of sea salt to milk to keep it fresh longer.
- **To set gelatin:** Place gelatin salads and desserts over ice sprinkled with sea salt to set quickly.

Raw Bee Products
Honey, I'm Home!

The most potent part of any plant is the flower, and the most potent part of the flower is the pollen. Pollen is roughly 35 percent predigested protein. This makes it easily assimilated for anyone with digestive issues. When digestion is weak, nearly all foods have a tendency to ferment and putrefy. That's why bee pollen and raw honey tonics are a wonderful solution for all cases of mild to moderate indigestion.

As an inverted sugar, bee pollen significantly boosts energy levels in the body because it allows the body to start burning essential fats for energy rather than burning sugars. Hence, bee pollen and honey are also considered excellent for the libido and for prostate health. Bee pollen also contains more digestible zinc than any other food. Zinc, an essential mineral that most people do not consume in adequate amounts, protects DNA from damage and promotes DNA repair. Furthermore, a study led by Emily Ho, PhD, at the Linus Pauling Institute confirms that a sufficient supply of zinc can help prevent prostate cancer. Chemical reactions with zinc often require copper and superoxide dismutase enzyme, both present in bee pollen.

Alain Callais, French agriculturalist and laureate of the Academy of Agriculture, believes that thirty-five grams of bee pollen per day satisfy all the necessary nutritional requirements of the average person. Twenty grams of bee pollen would constitute "a survival diet."[9] So, for pure good health and vitality, raw bee products—from royal jelly to propolis[10] to raw honey—are extraordinary as nutritional aids to help maintain and balance the diet.

Beauty and the Bees

I recommend that you always have bee pollen and raw honey on hand in your home. These wonderful natural substances can successfully treat insomnia, allergies, and fatigue, and help stave off the signs of aging. Always take bee pollen and raw, unfiltered honey together. Raw honey has antifungal, antiviral, and antibiotic properties. If you use bee pollen and raw honey consistently, as I do in my folk remedies at the Phoenix Institute, you will obtain the full spectrum of basic elements that the human body needs.

A natural sleeping tonic: Combine four tablespoons of raw honey, two teaspoons of bee pollen, and three teaspoons of apple cider vinegar in a cup of freshly boiled water. Sip slowly. This is a superb, all-natural sleep tonic.

Allergies and respiratory relief: Combine one tablespoon of raw honey, one teaspoon of bee pollen, and some lemon in one cup of freshly boiled water. This will soothe a sore throat, lungs in distress, or any other uncomfortable symptoms.

Oriental youth elixir: Combine two tablespoons of raw honey, two teaspoons of pollen, one-half cup of chopped ginseng, and dried orange peel. Eat with a spoon. The Chinese believe this combination creates a feeling of complete vitality and rejuvenation.

All-purpose body cream: Blend one peeled ripe banana, one peeled ripe avocado, and two teaspoons of bee pollen grains. This cream helps to reduce dryness, roughness, or wrinkles. Leave on the affected area

9 Carlson Wade, New Fact Book Bee Pollen and Your Health (Chicago, Keats Publishing).
10 Propolis is a natural antibiotic collected from the resinous mixture that honey bees gather from tree buds, sap flows, or other botanical sources.

for sixty minutes, then rinse. The cream can be stored in the refrigerator for up to two days.

All-purpose pollen lotion: To a cup of strained lemon juice, add one teaspoon of bee pollen and one-half cup of water. Keep refrigerated. Use for a facial, as a rinse, or as a shampoo additive for healthier hair. You can combine the lotion with other cosmetics as well.

Pollen youth bath: Fill a tub with warm water. Add one-half cup of bee pollen grains and a sliced fresh lemon. The lemon oils should release their enchanting fragrances and combine with the nectar scents of the pollen grains. Next, shine an ultraviolet flashlight on the bath water for two to five minutes. Then submerge yourself for thirty minutes. You will feel the invigorating effects. (Add two tablespoons of epsom salts or hydrogen peroxide for a stronger and more complete detoxification process.)

The Phoenix Institute Internal Tonic

I use this recipe for people with liver problems or digestive issues. It tastes delicious and can be taken a few times daily. The Phoenix Institute Internal Tonic will also benefit your immune and circulatory systems.

Ingredients:

2 tablespoons dried chopped comfrey root
1 tablespoon sassafras root bark

Boil one to four quarts of water, then let simmer for two to three hours. Then add two teaspoons of raw honey while the liquid is steaming to bring out the honey's beneficial compounds. Drink freely and enjoy.

Comfrey contains a substance called allantoin, a chemical compound proven to help cells grow and grow together. Although the U.S. Federal Drug Administration (FDA) has soured its reputation, comfrey has experienced centuries of success in healing and restoring bone and skin. Combined with a sweet, liver-boosting tonic such as sweet sassafras (the key ingredient in root beer) to help support the liver, this drink will boost your immune system and adaptogenic capacity. You should make at least one liter per person.

Did You Know?

Honey is a powerful preservative. Let a thirty-year-old jar of raw honey sit out in the sun and it will decrystallize and become a potent medicine once again. Is it any wonder some studies point out that beekeepers are the longest-living people in the world?

The following is a complete listing of all the nutrients found in bee pollen:

Vitamins

Provitamin A, thiamine, riboflavin, niacin, B6, pantothenic acid, biotin, B12, folic acid, choline, inositol, vitamin C, vitamin D, vitamin E, vitamin K, rutin

Minerals

Calcium, phosphorus, potassium, sulphur, sodium, chlorine, magnesium, iron, manganese, copper, iodine, zinc, manganese, silicon, molybdenum, boron, titanium

Enzymes

Amylase, diastase, saccharase, pectase, phosphatase, catalase, diaphorase, cozymase, cytochrome systems, lactic dehydrogenase, succinic dehydrogenase, 24 oxidoreductase, 21 transferases, 33 hydrolases, 11 lysases, 5 isomerases, pepsin, tryosin

Proteins and Amino Acids

Isoleucine, leucine, lysine, methionine, phenylalanine, threonine, tryptophan, valine, histidine, arginine, cystine, tyrosine, alanine, aspartic acid, glutamic acid, hydroxyproline, proline, serine

Others

Nucleic acids, flavonoids, phenolic acids, terpenes, nucleosides, auxins, fructose, glucose, brassins, gibberellins, kinins, verine, guanine, xanthine, lecithin, zeaxanthin, lycopene, hexadecanol, alpha-aminobutyric acid, monoglycerides, diglycerides, triglycerides, pentosans

Olive Oil
If it says Cold Pressed it's a Superfood

Cold-pressed olive oil is not chemically altered in any way.[11] It is nearly identical to human skin sebum. Its nutritious elements feed the brain and enhance the immune system. Drinking at least three tablespoons of cold-pressed olive oil every day can do wonders for your body and mind. Have you wondered why the Italians and Spanish are renowned for their beautiful skin, even in old age?

Olive oil oxygenates the skin and is a powerful healing force if regularly applied to the skin. It can be used to help fight infection of wounds and skin disease by simply applying it to the skin every other day. Olive oil has several key nutritional compounds, including:

- **Vitamin E**: An antioxidant that strengthens immune response and helps heal skin conditions. It contains essential fatty acids— good fats like omega-3 and omega-6—which improve brain function and organ health. Omega-3 and omega-6 taken in the right ratio can prevent sunburn.

---

11 In the Bible, Numbers 28:5 describes the broken olives that were placed in special baskets to collect the "first oil" or the "beaten oil." This was cold-pressed oil, unheated and unchanged in chemical structure, and used for its healing properties.

- **Chlorophyll:** This amazing antioxidant delivers some of the core nutritional minerals, such as magnesium and different nitrogen compounds.
- **Polyphenols:** These substances are also found in red wine and serve powerful antioxidant functions.
- **Phytoestrogens:** These substances help prevent bone loss and minimize irritating symptoms of menopause.

The Ancient Nutritionists

Long before modern nutritionists discovered the medicinal antibiotic properties of olive oil, Hippocrates used cold-pressed olive oil in over sixty different therapies. Olive oil—or as he called it, the "Great Therapeutic"—was prescribed for "diseases of women," skin rashes, mental illness, and oral hygiene. Hippocrates also recommended the process of oil pulling requires washing olive oil around the mouth for one minute and then spitting it back out. This type of oral cleansing is very effective in improving circulation as well as pulling out poisons that are lodged deep within the tissues of the mouth.

Aromatic lamps contained olive oil blended with rosemary or sage. In Greece, Rome, and Egypt, olive oil was infused with flowers and grasses to make beauty aids and various medicines. At the Phoenix Institute, we do the same thing today.

The Phoenix Institute's Mini Cold Infusion

A mini cold infusion is an old-fashioned way to produce high-quality essential oils from herbs. Any herb soaked in olive oil will eventually release large amounts of beneficial phytonutrients into the oil.

To make your own mini cold infusion:

Step 1: Inside a mason jar or jelly jar, combine rosemary and cinnamon with one cup of olive oil. Amounts of herbs may vary, but always allow enough olive oil to soak the tops of the herbs completely.

Step 2: Seal the jar tightly. Shake for three minutes every day for five days. Leave in the sunlight.

Step 3: On the fifth day, you will have a 12 percent essential oil blend of rosemary and cinnamon. Apply to bruised skin or rashes. Use within one month.

You can change up your mini cold infusion to disinfect cuts and bruises by using infused oregano oil. The antiseptic nature of oregano oil will heal cuts and bruises much faster.

For opening the lungs and improving digestion, use infused peppermint oil by applying it to the chest and lower back.

Do Not Underestimate the Benefits of Olive Oil

Professor Ancel Keys, an American scientist,[12] did research that showed a diet low in saturated fat and high in monosaturated fat might hold the secret to health and longevity. The beneficial effects of olive oil on blood cholesterol are already well-known. "Bad" cholesterol (LDL), a non-water soluble compound, can be lowered with significant amounts of olive oil rich in monosaturated fats. This is why olive oil is an excellent choice for circulation and heart health.

To add years to your life, get into the habit of drinking cold-pressed olive oil on a regular basis.[13]

- Lower your risk of heart disease and cancer
- Enhance your immune system
- Prevent cancer

---

12 http://en.wikipedia.org/wiki/Ancel_Keys.updated March 15, 2013.
13 Cal Orey. *The Healing Powers of Olive Oil: A Complete Guide to Nature's Liquid Gold.* January 29, 2008.

- Stave off diabetes
- Fight fat
- Slow the aging process

Did You Know?

- Olive oil also can be used to prevent rust by applying a light film to gardening tools.
- Mix a one-to-one ratio with vinegar to make a cleaning agent that does not smell, clears dust, and shines for a long time.

Colloidal Silver
The Silver Bullet

Silver was once used to ward off vampires. During the Black Plague, the wealthy classes used the antiviral properties of silver and garlic to protect themselves against infected people. During this time, children of wealth were given spoons made of pure silver to use for sucking and eating. This was seen as a way to combat infection, and thus the phrases "born with a silver spoon in his mouth" and "gets everything on a silver platter" were born.

The use of silver to treat wounds has significantly declined in the last one hundred years. This is the result of the publication in 1910 of the controversial Flexner Report, a comprehensive study of medical education written by Abraham Flexner under the auspices of the Carnegie Foundation. The Flexner Report is credited with helping to build the credibility of the American Medical Association while shutting down naturopathic schools and practitioners. In the naturopathic community, Flexner is notorious for his role in wiping out almost all botanical, homeopathic, osteopathic, and naturopathic schools by deeming them "unsafe." Colloidal silver was systematically removed from the United States Pharmacopeia after the release of the Flexner Report.[14]

---

14 Flexner Report, http://en.wikipedia.org/wiki/Flexner,updated July 2007.

Today, however, homeopathic-based medical treatments are returning: the silver-based salve, Silvadine, is used in virtually every burn ward in the US to kill infection, and the FDA has recently approved and licensed for sale a new silver-based bandage.

What Do They Know That We Don't?

- Silver water purification filters and tablets are manufactured in Switzerland for use in homes and offices. Many national and international airlines use them to prevent growth of algae and bacteria.
- Electrical ionization units that infuse water with silver and copper ions sanitize pool water without the harsh effects of chlorine in Switzerland.
- The former Soviet Union used silver to sterilize recycled water on their space vehicles.
- In the Japanese workplace, silver is a popular agent in the fight against airborne toxins as well as other industrial poisons.

How Best to Use Silver

Simply place colloidal silver into a spray bottle. You may cut it with colloidal copper or small amounts of colloidal gold as well. This silver spray has many wonderful applications because it is a natural disinfectant and antiseptic.

- Spray on anything from toothbrushes to eating utensils to safely sterilize them.
- Spray topically on cuts, wounds, abrasions, rashes, sunburn, insect bites, and bandages to prevent infection.
- Spray on Q-tips used for toenails, fingernails, and ear fungi.
- Mist kitchen sponges, towels, and cutting boards to eliminate E. coli and salmonella bacteria.
- Spray on garbage to prevent decay and odor.

- Spray your refrigerator, freezer, and the insides of food storage bins.
- Spray pet bedding and let dry to disinfect.
- Spray on the tops of opened jam, jelly, and condiment containers, and inside the jar and inside the lid before replacing.
- Spray on toilet seats, bowls, tile floors, sinks, urinals, and doorknobs.
- Spray on diapers to prevent diaper rash.
- Spray in the air to prevent the spread of colds, flu, pneumonia, staph, strep, respiratory infections, and rhinoviruses, and to speed recovery.
- Spray and wipe telephone mouthpieces, headphones, hearing aids, eyeglass frames, hairbrushes, and combs,
- Spray and add to sprouting seed water or soaking waters to retard decay and odor, and to promote fantastic sprout freshness.
- Spray on fruits and vegetables to remove pesticides and other harmful elements, and then rinse.
- Spray into suspect drinking water when traveling or camping.

Thanks to the Trinity College of Natural Health for compiling the list below of medical conditions seen to benefit from colloidal silver prior to 1938:

Acne
Adenovirus
Aspergillus niger
Athlete's foot
Anthrax bacillus
Appendicitis
Axillae and blind boils of the neck
Bacillus typhus
B. coli
B. coli communis
B. dysenteriae
B. pyocyaneus
B. tuberculosis
Bacillary dysentery
Biological weapons bladder irritation
Blepharitis
Boils
Bovine rotavirus
Bromidrosis in axillae
Bromidrosis in feet
Bronchitis
Burns and wounds of the cornea
Bladder infection
Candida albicans (yeast infection)
Chronic cystitis

Chronic eczema of the anterior nares
Chronic eczema of metus of ear
Colitis
Conjunctivitis (pink eye)
Corneal infection ulcers
Cystitis
Dacryocystitis
Dandruff
Dental abscess/infection, caries
Dermatitis suggestive of toxemia
Diarrhea
Diphtheria
Dysentery
Ear affections
E. coli
Entamoeba histolytica (cysts)
Enlarged prostate
Epididymitis
Erysipelas
Escherichia coli
Eustachian tubes (potency restored)
Fever
Follicular tonsillitis
Furunculosis
Gonococcus
Gonorrhea
Hemorrhoids
Hepatitis
Herpetic whitlow (herpes)
Hypopyon ulcer
Impetigo
Infantile disease
Infected ulcers of the cornea
Inflammatory rheumatism
Infection
Influenza (flu)
Interstitial keratitis
Intestinal troubles
Jock itch
Karposi's sarcoma
Legionella pneumophila
Lesion healing
Leucorrhoea vaginal yeast
Meniere's symptoms
Meningitis
MRSA
Nasopharyngeal catarrh (reduced)
Offensive discharge of chronic suppuration in otitis media
Ophthalmic practices
Osteomalacia
Paramecium
Parathyroid
Perineal eczema
Phlegmons
Phlyctenular conjunctivitis
Pneumonia
Polio virus 1
Pruritus ani
Pseudomonas aeruginosa
Puerperal septicemia
Quinsy rhinitis
Ringworm of the body
Salmonella
Scarlatina
Sepsis
Septic tonsillitis
Septic ulcers of the legs
Shingles
Sinusitis
Soft sores
Spore forming bacteria

Spring catarrh
Sprue
Staphylolysin (Inhibits)
Staphylococcus aureus (including MR strains)
Streptococci
Strep virus
Tinea versicolor

Typhoid
Typhoid bacillus
Ulcerative Urticaria
Urticaria suggestive of toxemia
Vaginal discharge
Vegetative B cereus cells
Vincent's angina
Vorticellae
Warts
Whooping cough

Castor Oil
A Versatile Remedy

Castor oil, which comes from the palma Christi plant (hand of Christ plant), is a unique antibiotic and anti-inflammatory. A radical hydrogen compound built into its chemical structure gives it a magnetic quality so that castor oil has a "live wire" nature. Because of this quality, castor oil mirrors and thus supports the electrical nature of the body. Plus, it contains high levels of vitamin E and antioxidants, and has circulation-enhancing emollient properties. I highly recommend castor oil as another tool in your holistic health medicine chest.

Castor oil is an extremely powerful purgative. Edgar Cayce, often called the father of holistic medicine, recommended castor oil at over one thousand of his readings. Where ingesting castor oil could be of some benefit (for example a strong need to cleanse the body quickly), I recommend one-eighth to one-quarter teaspoon of castor oil, followed with a glass or two of distilled water to help flush internal toxic debris. Before you try this remedy, please consult your doctor or health care practitioner.

Researchers have demonstrated that castor oil increases lymphocytes when applied to the liver, improving the immune system. We know that it can potentially eliminate cancerous legions because there are hundreds, if not thousands, of reported cases of this occurring. We know castor oil increases the alkalinity of the system. We know that castor oil, when applied to the navel, can increase libido. Ancient and modern chinese medicine is rich with tales of castor oil's healing prowess. Throughout human history, castor oil has been proven safe and effective for thousands of years. Yet ironically, we are still not sure how it works chemically on the body.

Nonetheless, it does work. To use castor oil topically, heat one tablespoon of castor oil over a stove until it is warm. While it is warm, apply some to the desired part of your body. I strongly recommend applying castor oil to your liver/solar plexus region. Gently massage the oil into your body for 100-600 strokes. This will provide you with castor oil's general health promoting effects. I also recommend you wear a white cotton shirt after applying castor oil to your body. This will help the castor oil work its way into your body and will prevent your outer clothes from getting oiled.

Health and Beauty Uses

Castor oil is highly electrical and soothing, with powerful healing properties. Because of its versatility, it can be applied externally to any area of the body. You may use castor oil at room temperature, or heat it over a stove in a spoon, and apply it externally to any problem area. Here are some suggestions for using castor oil to improve your well-being and appearance:

- If you have a lot of fat around the belly button, apply castor oil to burn acids in the system and burn body fat in a very short time.
- If you have dermatitis, especially any skin infection or rash, apply castor oil directly onto the affected area.
- For muscle sprains or a stiff neck, apply castor oil and massage into the skin.
- Use castor oil under the eyes to improve the elasticity of skin and reduce wrinkles. You don't have to pay hundreds of dollars for sophisticated beauty creams; a dab of clean, golden castor oil will do the job.

"Glyco"
A Forgotten Jewel

Glycothymoline (Glyco) is a long-forgotten health jewel. Fifty years ago, people commonly used it as a mouthwash and antiseptic. I recommend it as an alkaline-cleansing solution of the first order, and as a treatment for arthritis, excess mucus, headaches, and much more. Today, however, it is only available on the Internet, but is inexpensive.

Glyco becomes more powerful when used as a Glyco pack, frequently recommended for osteoarthritis, burns, rashes, and virtually all conditions of the skin. Glyco packs can aid circulation, promote muscle relaxation, relieve inflammation, and supply moisture. To use as a pack, soak cotton flannel or regular gauze with Glyco and wrap the area of soreness. If you add sea salt to the gauze and apply heat to the affected area, the soreness will begin to subside.

According to Edgar Cayce, a few drops of Glyco in water acts as an intestinal antiseptic. He claimed that it helps the body form pepsins, which in turn keep the body's systems much more alkaline. He also recommended taking three drops in water before bedtime.[15]

15 Cayce Health Data Banks, Cecil Nichols. http://www.edgarcayce.org/are/holistic health/data/thglyco1.html, March 1966.

Glyco-Tiger Protocol

At the Phoenix Institute, we have found great success using Glyco and castor oil together.[16] Our Glyco-Tiger Protocol treats respiratory ailments by removing mucus and thoroughly alkalinizing the body's systems. This protocol relieves cold symptoms, opens up the lungs and respiratory passages, and enhances mood.

To experience the full benefits of the Glyco-Tiger Protocol, I recommend you take the following steps:

Step 1: Wash your mouth for three minutes with three tablespoons of Glyco combined with three tablespoons of hydrogen peroxide.

Step 2: Apply castor oil to the middle abdomen.

Step 3: Apply regular Tiger Balm, a popular salve that can be purchased at your local drugstore, to the chest.

Step 4: Rinse both hands in Glyco while breathing deeply. Let your hands dry for five minutes.

Step 5: Drink three tablespoons of cold-pressed olive oil.

Step 6: After 10 minutes, drink two glasses of lemon water.

The dynamic combination of Glyco and castor oil will help to clear your gastro-intestinal system. You will feel refreshed, relaxed, and in radiant health.

---

16 Thanks to Edgar Cayce. Ibid.

The Black Scarf

Sleep is the most important component of physical health. Over exposure to light at work and home has resulted in an epidemic imbalance of serotonin, a major neurotransmitter responsible for feelings of well-being and happiness. Many people report having trouble sleeping; some people do not sleep deep enough, while others sleep, but wake up tired. Using a black scarf with earplugs can help restore serotonin balance and help you consciously relax, and sleep.

Releasing the Sleep Hormone

Did you ever have something pressing on your mind that you could not stop thinking about? I think we all have. In fact, this type of distracted mental behavior, commonly called "monkey mind," is believed to be rooted in the depravity of the human and spiritual condition. From Australia to India, yogis working to attain mastery over their physical bodies and senses are put to the test in dark caves for a series of days, or even weeks. In addition to their prescribed meditative disciplines, they experience a darkness and silence that literally banishes all distractions and forces their bodies into long periods of dreamtime (a theta/delta brain wave pattern or melatonin-dominant state). In this state, the body releases a powerful cascade of the healing sleep hormone, melatonin.

Melatonin's flow controls how deeply you sleep, how long you sleep, and how well the body repairs itself. It also serves as a powerful antidepressant and antioxidant, with fantastic anti-aging and disease-preventing properties. Melatonin is produced primarily in the pineal gland, but is also produced in the retina and the gastrointestinal tract. It is the ultimate restorative hormone. In conjuring up any healing protocol, it is worth taking advantage of its powers. Best of all, you can obtain it naturally—from your brain, your eyes, and your gut.

Melatonin also can help to significantly decrease "bad" cholesterol (LDL) and increase "good" cholesterol (HDL) levels. According to Professor A. Wakatsuki in the *Journal of Pineal Research* 2008, heart disease is still the leading cause of death in the United States and so enhancing your production of melatonin has real health benefits. Studies conducted by Dr. Reiter as reported in the September, 2012 issue of *Life Extension* magazine indicate that in some cases, melatonin is six times more powerful than L- glutathione, an antioxidant with a long list of proven medical values. Dr. Reiter also noted that melatonin is useful to help prevent Alzheimer's disease, obesity, and osteoporosis.

I also suggest eating enough almonds, beets, mustard, cucumbers, tomatoes, turkey, and bananas. These foods all contain melatonin's amino-acid derivative, L-tryptophan, which helps to foster sleepiness. Now to the black scarf.

The Black Scarf

To replicate the yogis' experience in the cave, try using a blindfold to help balance your brain chemistry, improve your concentration, and produce better quality sleep. I recommend using a black scarf for this purpose. It is an excellent addition to a meditation or contemplation practice

Blindfolded Basic Relaxation Exercise

Let's get started. Sit on a pillow. Place your scarf or blinders over your head and wear earplugs. Relax every muscle in your body.

Inhale deeply while counting backward from seven. Hold your breath for four seconds and focus on the feeling of supreme comfort. Then exhale slowly for eight seconds. Continue with this seven-four-eight breath count. You may do this sixty times, or for no more than forty-five minutes.

Afterward, lie down and relax. You should easily fall asleep.

Blindfolded Yoga

Yoga helps to circulate blood and energy through the brain and into the rest of the body. Blindfolded yoga helps strengthen your nervous system, determination, and mental acuity. By practicing yoga blindfolded and with earplugs, breathing slowly and deeply, and staying attentive and relaxed, you will find that in fifteen minutes you will flush your brain with melatonin-rich blood. This will make for a powerful practice. Be sure you do enough forward bends and inversions to facilitate this process even more.

You may find this practice more difficult than normal because your nervous system will not be used to working in a dreamtime state.

Blindfolded Exercise

Essentially any exercise that enables you to breathe while staying in a single location is worth practicing blindfolded. I prefer qigong and jumping jacks. Jumping jacks are wonderful to do with a blindfold because they help increase circulation and offer a full range of motion. Qigong lifts the spirits and facilitates power breathing. Try jumping jacks for five minutes, then qigong for fifteen minutes with your earplugs in and blinders down. Continue to breathe with rhythm, consciously and evenly. You will feel awesome.

Another Use for Your Black Scarf

Eye masks tend to fall off at night and do not filter out all the light. A black scarf is more workable for this purpose. For deeper sleep, wrap a black scarf around your eyes. This will balance serotonin and produce melatonin in the brain all night. I recommend using it at night and for an hour during the day. This will assist with your contemplation, meditation, or limbic breathing practices.

Before going to sleep at night, I also recommend that you put on your black scarf and walk around your room blindfolded as an exercise. This can produce more melatonin. Just as important, it engenders trust in yourself. Be open to the idea that you can breathe deeply while walking blindly around your room. Remember to catalyze the process; breathe, breathe, and breathe some more.[17]

---

17 http://www.lef.org/magazine/mag2012/sep2012_7-Ways-Melatonin-Attacks-Aging-Factors_01.htm.

Activated Charcoal
Earth, Wind, and Fire

Activated charcoal has traditionally been used to treat food poisoning, intestinal issues, flatulence, and stomach cramps. However, most of its healing applications are not common knowledge today. What makes activated charcoal such a superb medicine? Under a very fine microscope, you will see what looks like a series of caverns. The openings in these caverns sometimes measure no larger than several nanometers, larger than some viruses. As a result, charcoal has an amazing ability to trap unwanted viruses, bacteria, toxins, and everyday pollutants.

Underappreciated Charcoal Use

Charcoal is without a doubt the most underappreciated substance in the United States. Nuclear submarines use charcoal to remove carbon dioxide from the air to enable breathing; space stations and water and air purification systems use it, too. Charcoal can also neutralize mustard gas, anthrax, and other chemical warfare agents. Charcoal is used as a top dressing for gardens and lawns. It sweetens the soil and neutralizes pesticides and herbicides. Soaps, oils, and a myriad of other everyday products contain charcoal as a preservative and detergent. Charcoal is used in the production of silk, and is the preferred tool of Japanese sumi-e art. It is used to recover and extract gold on a large, industrial scale. And the food industry uses charcoal to clean obnoxious odors, flavors, or unwanted pigments from many foods, including cooking oils.

So charcoal purifies our water, filters air, cleans our food, and helps us make the clothes we wear. We grow our food and foliage in it, go to war with it, and take it with us into the depths of the oceans and into space. We paint with charcoal, and we use it to help us clean up messes. Even trees scarred by old forest fires tend to live much longer because their blackened bark has become germicidal, preventing rot from occurring within the tree.

Charcoal has antibacterial and antifungal properties. It is a proven liver detoxifier, helps to restore bowel health, and supports the growth of friendly flora in the intestine. Amazingly, charcoal is very body friendly and can pass right through the gastro-intestinal tract without a problem.

"Wood Feeds Fire; Fire Creates Earth; Earth Bears Metal; Metal Carries Water"

This Chinese school of thought teaches that the five phases of nature correspond to their five seasons of the calendar. Just like spring, summer, late summer, fall, and winter make up their five seasons, water, fire, metal, wood, and earth comprise the five phases of nature. Throughout the year, water extinguishes fire, fire melts metal, metal chops wood, wood parts the earth (think of tree roots), and earth dams water.

Early in recorded history, Chinese medicine had developed a complete system of healing. In fact, medical researchers today survey the body with high tech receivers to pick up electrical channels that the Chinese termed "meridians" around 3000 BC. Not only did the Chinese have a working system of medicine and health thousands of years ago, but they also sought to understand and harmonize health with the movements of nature. It is important to note that the use of activated charcoal was very popular in ancient China. Why? Ask yourself how activated charcoal is created. It is born from earth, charred by fire, boiled in water, cooled in air and then powdered. It truly embodies the phases of earth, wood, wind, and fire. No wonder it is renowned for its marvelous qualities as a medicine.

Health and Beauty Uses

Though thousands of uses exist for this unattractive, blackish-brown substance, I will list only a few here.

Compress: As a compress, activated charcoal treats ulcers, food poisoning, liver damage, jaundice, injuries, broken bones, fingernail fungus, candidiasis, appendicitis, diabetes, cancer, and much more. Combine charcoal compresses with flaxseed or slippery elm bark to help deliver the charcoal into the body.

Hot Footbath: I highly recommend the hot footbath method, another popular use for charcoal that uses heat to further activate charcoal's restorative properties. In a basin, combine hot water and approximately five tablespoons of activated charcoal. Place your feet in the water for forty minutes. You may also add one ounce of hydrogen peroxide. This will help relieve fatigue and muscle soreness.

Regular Hot Bath: For general health and to disperse ionizing radiation, soak for twenty minutes to one hour in a hot bath with one-half cup of activated charcoal. You will sweat out many toxins because of the detoxification properties of charcoal.

Toothpaste: Add a pinch of activated charcoal to your toothpaste to disinfect your mouth and whiten your teeth.

Stomachaches: Place activated charcoal powder into capsules that you can buy at your pharmacy or online. Take one to three capsules for mild to severe stomachaches, light detoxification, or for your daily health maintenance needs.

Facial/skin mask: Charcoal prevents the decay of tissue, making it an effective antiwrinkle treatment, so add activated charcoal to face cream to create an excellent beauty mask. Activated charcoal added to body lotion also works well as a topical ointment to treat poison ivy, bug bites, or rashes.

The Infrared Pollen Charcoal Bath

This remedy is excellent for a full-body detox. You will need activated charcoal, bee pollen, and an infrared heat lamp.

Why add bee pollen?

As we have explained, bee pollen is a complete, disease-fighting, vitamin-abundant nutrient that positively affects premature aging, digestive upsets, prostate diseases, sore throats, acne, fatigue, sexual problems, allergies, and many other conditions. Add it to a bath to make it more restorative.

How does an infrared heat lamp work?

Infrared light and heat are classified as medical devices in Canada and Japan. Infrared heat vibrates at the same speed as water molecules. Infrared heat lamps also promote circulation and heat shock proteins (current research indicates that heat shock proteins may be powerful immune-system builders). You will find many benefits to having your own infrared heat lamp, activated charcoal, and an ample supply of bee pollen in your bathroom.

Instructions

1. Purchase an infrared heat lamp, or Designers Edge E-240 incandescent brooder light fitted with a GE 37771 R40 250-watt red heat lamp. These have been tested to operate at the proper far-infrared spectrum.
2. Fill a tub with hot water and add one-third cup of activated charcoal. Wait for one hour as the water purifies. After thirty minutes, shine the heat lamp on the water.

3. When the water is sufficiently hot, add one-half to three-quarters cup of bee pollen granules. Slice three or four lemons and throw them into the bath as well.
4. Soak for thirty to forty minutes and enjoy.

Note: Lemon oils will release aromatic compounds inside the bee pollen. The bath will smell like a lush forest of flowers on a beautiful midsummer's eve.

The Activated Charcoal Peroxide Bath

Activated charcoal and hydrogen peroxide combined will get you clean, rejuvenated, detoxified, and energized. While activated charcoal cleans, hydrogen peroxide oxygenates. While charcoal brings circulation, hydrogen peroxide stabilizes blood chemistry. The activated charcoal and hydrogen peroxide bath is one of my favorite holistic health techniques. Think of the activated charcoal peroxide bath as rain falling on burning wood. What a natural way to sooth the inner fires and strengthen the vitality of the body's ecosystem!

Use one-third cup of peroxide and an equal amount of activated charcoal powder. Add the charcoal and hydrogen peroxide to hot water. Soak, relax, and enjoy.

The High-Frequency Violet Ray
Back to the Future

Meet Nikola Tesla, the indisputable father of robotics, AC power, the X-ray, and the radio.[18] This singular visionary scientist created the high-frequency violet-ray healing device designed to sterilize water and food, clean the air, fertilize the soil, and heal a host of human ailments. Today, his influence should be noted with every flick of a light switch. He intended his high-frequency healing devices to enable future generations to clean and ionize air and water, sterilize food, fertilize soil with nitrogen compounds, and heal their bodies.[19] With his message of world peace, his dream still holds many possibilities.

---

18 Nikola Tesla is the unsung progenitor of the radio and X-ray. Tesla, on hearing of Marconi's efforts, is said to have remarked to a friend, "Marconi is a good fellow. Let him continue. He is using seventeen of my patents." Margaret Cheney, *Tesla: Man Out of Time,* (Oct. 2, 2001). See also, *My Inventions,* (New York City, Nikola Tesla Hart Bros. Publishing).

19 Ibid.

Did You Have Any Idea?

In 1910, ozone-generating systems were in high demand. Most people who could afford them had heard of them, used them, or purchased them. They were often used in beauty parlors and doctor's offices. Yet hardly anyone has heard of them today, and most who have do not know what purpose they served.

The high-frequency violet ray's therapeutic action at the biological level comes from the unit's electrical current, which is discharged between the electrode and the body surface. This device consists of a Tesla coil attached to a vacuum tube containing either argon or neon gas. A high-frequency current is fired into the tube, passes through the glass, and transforms the surrounding air, resulting in pure oxygen, ozone, nitric oxide, and other gases. These vital gases are then transferred through the skin via the high-frequency current. Our skin safely conducts this particular type of current. It works ingeniously. I have seen these devises heal skin rashes, muscle cramps, headaches, and even balding!

Oxygen, Nitrogen, and Ozone: The Royal Heirs of the Body

To truly understand the benefits of a high-frequency violet ray machine, you must first understand the value of oxygen, nitrogen, and ozone. The body can only use activated oxygen. When oxygen enters a healthy body, it splits apart and becomes "activated" when an electron attaches to it. It then forms other oxygen compounds, such as nitric oxide, singlet oxygen, hydrogen peroxide, and ozone, which clean the cells of the body. Dirty cells cannot function properly, making oxygen metabolism the most important aspect of chemistry related to body health. A high-frequency violet ray device delivers activated oxygen in all of its forms.

The body also needs a balance of nitrogen and oxygen. The high-frequency violet ray machine helps fix nitrogen into the body while enabling a more efficient use of oxygen. Our bodies especially need to receive balanced portions of nitrogen and oxygen in our sleeping environments. Therefore, it's important to ensure that we breathe clean air with ample parts nitrogen and oxygen. I highly recommend keeping a few plants in your bedroom for this purpose. In the back of this book, you will find information on Six Air Purifying House Plants that I think do the trick.

If we breathe in too much carbon dioxide, the oxygen in our bodies can become poisonous, a condition known in the scientific community as oxygen toxicity. As a result, human beings instinctively try to metabolize this overabundance of poisoned oxygen by consuming large quantities of iron-based foods. This causes large accumulations of iron in the body, even on the cellular level. Because of an overabundance of carbon dioxide in the air, we have an overabundance of iron in the body. Heavy metal detoxification is therefore a top priority in any health regime. High-frequency violet ray devices can help with localized areas of iron overabundance in the brain, the palms of the hands, and the bottoms of the feet.

We also all need ozone, which has a long, impressive history of healing all manner of infirmities. Of all the oxygen compounds that benefit the body, ozone is perhaps the best. The body itself produces its own form of ozone, called ozonide. In its natural form, ozone can clean the air and has been reputed to reverse Lyme disease, and even cancer.[20]

Let's Get Technical

The therapeutic action of a high-frequency violet ray machine lies in five important qualities:

1. A wide band of electromagnetic radiation (from the supersonic to the ultraviolet spectrum)
2. The high-frequency current flowing through tissue depths
3. The thermal radiation arising in the tissues and in the unit discharge field

20 Gary Null, *Ozone Therapy: The Miracle Medicine.*(New York City, Gary Null Associates, 2007)(DVD).

4. The weak-intensity ultrasonic vibrations arising directly in tissues (oscillation effect)
5. Chemically active substances—ozone, nitric oxides, and singlet oxygen—in small but significant amounts

High-frequency violet ray machines deliver activated oxygen in all of its forms, producing ozone and nitric oxide and delivering all these gases through the capillaries into the blood. In water, it can create hydrogen peroxide. It also cleans the air of carbon-based pollution, and is very effective in dealing with EMF (electromagnetic field) overexposure.

Suggestions, Suggestions, Suggestions

High-frequency violet ray machines are particularly useful for warts, baldness, wrinkles, skin tone, and skin elasticity. I encourage you to use one by placing the wand at the top of your head, as you would a brush or a comb, and slowly moving it down the spine.[21] You can use it right before bed to improve the quality of your sleep. Consuming vitamin C and large amounts of raw, chlorophyll-rich foods can make your oxygen metabolism much more efficient, especially in conjunction with a high-frequency treatment, with cumulative effects. I prefer to use the high-frequency violet ray device in the morning—for no more than fifteen minutes—on the scalp, face, and neck after gargling hydrogen peroxide for at least one minute.

Use a high-frequency violet ray over your food as an effective way to energize and sterilize your meals. It is chemical-free and residue-free, can sterilize cuts, and works well on sprains, rashes, sores, cuts, aches, bumps, and systemic conditions. High-frequency violet ray devices can remove odors from the home. No other device can purify water, cleanse food, and clean the air at home. This is the technology of the future.

---

21 High-frequency violet ray machines may be purchased at the Phoenix Institute.

Basic Guidelines for Using the High-Frequency Violet Ray Device

Always unplug and disassemble the unit after using it. Keep it in a dry place. Humidity will temporarily disable the unit.

- Use the device for no more than twenty minutes at a time.
- Always press very firmly on the body and move the tube over the surface very slowly.
- Rinse the glass electrode tube with hydrogen peroxide or alcohol after using.
- Sterilize food and clean water with the far end of the tube.

While soaking your feet in hydrogen peroxide footbath, use the high-frequency violet ray on the top of the head, back of the neck and the spine. Afterward, apply castor oil to sensitive areas. Castor oil maintains superb electrical balance when rubbed on tissues following a high-frequency violet ray treatment.

Be careful not to turn the high-frequency violet ray up to high intensity immediately after turning it on. It must first warm up. Not allowing a warm-up period may cause a shock to the body.

Chlorophyll Pollen
36-Hour Fast

A Complete-Meal Smoothie Fast, Specifically
Designed to Reduce Food Cravings

Instructions

After you have gathered a few of the items discussed in this book, I invite you to put them to use. This Chlorophyll Pollen Fast is a wonderful project for those looking to lose weight, increase energy and improve overall health.

Day 1

At no later than 2:00 p.m., enjoy a large, healthy, organic soup. It should contain whole grains, vegetables, and protein components. This soup should contain *no* allergens such as gluten or dairy. Chicken soup, lentil soup, black bean soup, and wild rice with fish soup are all acceptable. This will be the last meal of the day, so make it large and healthy.

At 7:00 p.m. prepare an Ali's Shake:

> 2 heaping tablespoons of lecithin granules
> 2 heaping tablespoons of ground flaxseed
> 3 heaping tablespoons of protein powder*

In a blender, blend in 32 oz. of water, 1 cup of dandelions, kale, lettuce, or broccoli
*Hemp, whey, or even egg protein powders are acceptable.

The Bee Pollen and Vinegar Sleepy Time Tonic

Before bed, bring a fresh pot of water to a boil. Add three tablespoons of apple cider vinegar, two teaspoons of bee pollen, two teaspoons of raw honey, and a dash of cinnamon to a large cup of hot water. Drink at least one cup and go to sleep.

Day 2

Begin this day with twelve deep breaths, a glass of distilled water, some optional dance, light stretching, or exercise. Play beautiful music, and then take a hot, conventional, 3-percent hydrogen peroxide bath. Stay in the bath no longer than thirty minutes.

Hydrogen Peroxide Bath Instructions

Add one-half cup of hydrogen peroxide to hot bath water with equal amounts of charcoal, epsom salt, and apple cider vinegar.

At 10:00 a.m., make a Bee Pollen Breakfast Blend

Begin your day with this complete protein beverage. The Bee Pollen Breakfast Blend is specifically designed to eliminate food cravings.

Bring at least 32 ounces of purified water to a boil. Add:

3 tablespoons bee pollen
2 tablespoons raw honey
2 juiced lemons
Small pinch of saffron

Important: After you finish this drink, enjoy three tablespoons of coconut oil within a period of fifteen minutes. Then go for a nice walk.

At 12:00 p.m., make a Blue Nut Milk Smoothie:

(If you do not feel like drinking a smoothie, then skip this step.)

Blend five almonds and five blueberries in at least 32 oz. of filtered water. Continue as if preparing Ali's Shake.

Important: Between 12:30 and 5:00 p.m., drink at least four tablespoons of cold-pressed olive oil. Take another nice walk.

At Sunset: Prepare another Ali's Shake. Add two teaspoons of bee pollen and raw honey to this Shake. Also, use a different protein powder then you used before, if possible.

Afterward, prepare two cups of hot saffron tea. Drink outside and take plenty of deep breaths. Saffron tea has been proven to balance brain chemistry and significantly decrease cravings.

Remember: Use no more than a pinch of saffron in each cup. If your food cravings persist, I advise drinking another Sleepy Time Tonic.

Day 3

Before breakfast, follow the morning instructions for Day 2. Then, prepare one last Bee Pollen Breakfast Blend.

An excellent 'Breaking the Fast' meal:

Eat a large organic leafy salad. Then cook one small bowl of GMO-free polenta with clarified butter or cold-pressed olive oil. You may add one organic cage free egg and/or a mixture of raw nuts and seeds if you desire. Enjoy the rest of your day!

SIX AIR PURIFYING HOUSE PLANTS

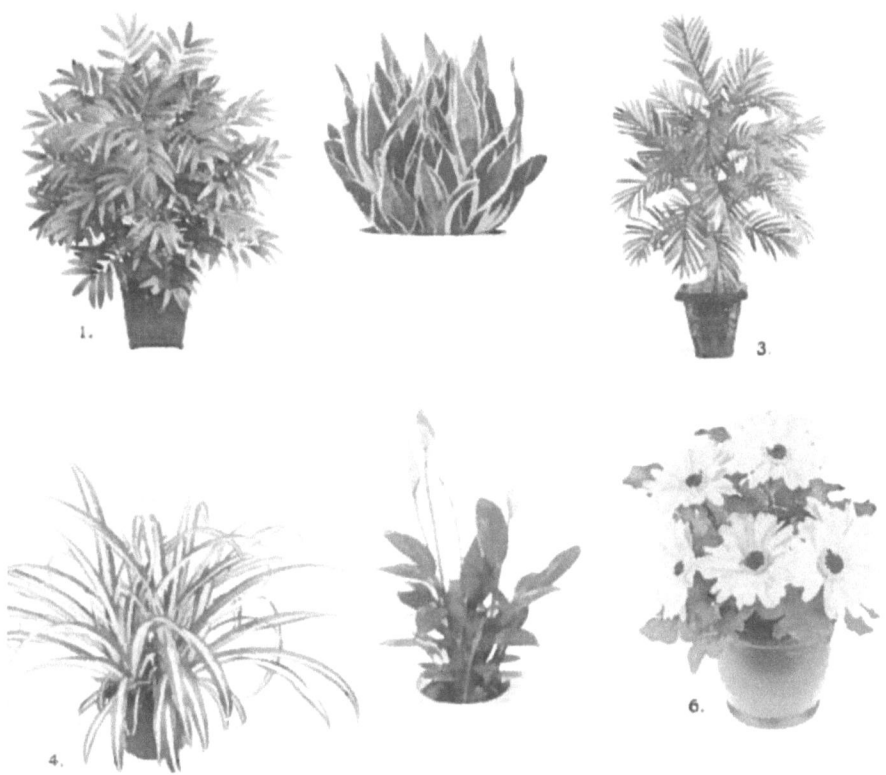

1. **Bamboo Palm:** According to NASA, it removes formaldehyde and is said to act as a natural humidifier.
2. **Snake Plant:** Found by NASA to absorb nitrogen oxides and formaldehyde.

3. **Areca Palm:** One of the best air-purifying plants for general air cleanliness.

4. **Spider Plant:** A great Indoor plant for removing carbon monoxide and other toxins or impurities. Spider plants are one of three plants NASA deems best at removing formaldehyde from the air.

5. **Peace Lily:** Peace lilies could be called the "clean-all." They are often placed in bathrooms or laundry rooms because they are known to remove mold spores as well as formaldehyde and trichloroethylene.

6. **Gerbera Daisy:** Not only do these gorgeous flowers remove benzene from the air, they are known to improve sleep by absorbing carbon dioxide and giving off more oxygen at night than during the day.

About Me

I was raised in a health-conscious family. My mother placed emphasis on conventional education *and* personal freedom. My father taught me how to ignore the world in order to follow my dreams. Through my teenage years, I suffered from undiagnosed Epstein Barr syndrome, chronic fatigue, years of chronic primary insomnia, constant throat, ear, and skin infection, and ultimately a full-blown case of shingles. At eighteen, my shingles transformed into an uncomfortable case of long-term post-herpetic neuralgia—a nerve condition felt in the arms and throat. As a result of my condition, I could no longer articulate certain sounds. My hands and arms, sometimes paralyzed, always felt pain. I dropped out of school. Defeated in body and soul, I passed the time reading books in my room. While reading, living in my own world for over three years with old jazz and blues records, I licked my wounds and discovered I had nothing to lose.

My first landmark change was to stop abusing my mind with television. After that, I stopped abusing my body with medication. At twenty-one, I began to fast, diet, practice yoga, and zealously research the health sciences. I found observing my own healing sobering and incredibly liberating. Naturally, I sought to improve other areas of my life. As time went by, I gained many rich experiences in recovery and personal healing.

More than anything, I still desire to learn from the irreverent wisdom of my twenty-one-year-old self; a young man who found it so incredibly easy to release himself from his past and walk toward a brighter unknown. When I am gone, this is how I would like to be known. I am a graduate, health educator, and recognized speaker of the Hippocrates Health Institute, as well as a Certified Natural Health Professional (CNHP) by the Trinity College of Natural Health. I teach workshops on health, sustainability, and disaster preparedness. I have reversed my long-term, post-herpetic neuralgia, a known "irreversible" nervous system condition. I have enjoyed my first unmedicated sleep in seven years. Today I proudly manage a holistic healing center, The Phoenix Institute of Holistic Health and Research, in Montclair, New Jersey. I am politically active and support the empowerment of all people.

www.ingramcontent.com/pod-product-compliance
Lightning Source LLC
Chambersburg PA
CBHW020902310526
45786CB00018B/1530